THE CARRIAGE RIDE

OR

QUITE POSSIBLY THE JOURNEY OF YOUR LIFE

JACQUIE ROBINSON

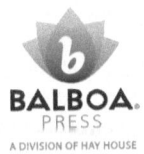

BALBOA
PRESS
A DIVISION OF HAY HOUSE

Copyright © 2016 Jacquie Robinson.

All rights reserved. No part of this book may be used or reproduced by any means, graphic, electronic, or mechanical, including photocopying, recording, taping or by any information storage retrieval system without the written permission of the author except in the case of brief quotations embodied in critical articles and reviews.

Balboa Press books may be ordered through booksellers or by contacting:

Balboa Press
A Division of Hay House
1663 Liberty Drive
Bloomington, IN 47403
www.balboapress.com.au
1 (877) 407-4847

Because of the dynamic nature of the Internet, any web addresses or links contained in this book may have changed since publication and may no longer be valid. The views expressed in this work are solely those of the author and do not necessarily reflect the views of the publisher, and the publisher hereby disclaims any responsibility for them.

The author of this book does not dispense medical advice or prescribe the use of any technique as a form of treatment for physical, emotional, or medical problems without the advice of a physician, either directly or indirectly. The intent of the author is only to offer information of a general nature to help you in your quest for emotional and spiritual well-being. In the event you use any of the information in this book for yourself, which is your constitutional right, the author and the publisher assume no responsibility for your actions.

Any people depicted in stock imagery provided by Thinkstock are models, and such images are being used for illustrative purposes only.
Certain stock imagery © Thinkstock.

This workbook is designed to provide knowledge through a self-reflective study experience. It can be used to assist individual and group therapy sessions.

Print information available on the last page.

ISBN: 978-1-5043-0298-2 (sc)
ISBN: 978-1-5043-0299-9 (e)

Balboa Press rev. date: 07/07/2016

Contents

The Carriage Ride: A Guide to Understanding Yourself ix

The Ride of Your Life Workbook x

The Ride of Your Life Model xii

The Carriage 1

The Horse 10

The Driver 17

The Master—The Inner Self 34

The Road 40

LIST OF EXERCISES

Exercise 1: To Start xi

Exercise 2: Family Tree 3

Exercise 3: Carriage Care 6

Exercise 4: Physical Fitness 7

Exercise 5: Horse-Drawn Carriages 8

Exercise 6: Horse Breeds 15

Exercise 7: You Make Me Feel 20

Exercise 8: Distinguish Your Thoughts from Your Feelings 22

Exercise 9: Life is Not Fair 29

Exercise 10: Self-Talk 33

Exercise 11: Describing the Master 38

Exercise 12: Draw a Road 41

Exercise 13: Probing Your Life's Journey 42

Exercise 14: Storyboard 43

Exercise 15: Dot-to-Dot Road Map 44

Exercise 16: The Three Ss and Two Ts 46

Exercise 17: Obstacles 50

Exercise 18: Doubts, Fears, and Worries 55

Exercise 19: The Famous Five Ws 57

Exercise 20: Using the Model to Master Your Life 61

THE CARRIAGE RIDE
A GUIDE TO UNDERSTANDING YOURSELF

This workbook is designed to be read with a pencil in hand. It is an excellent workbook for self-study as well as individual and group therapy learning. All material is copyright-protected and cannot be duplicated without permission from the publisher. Therefore, be sure to order a copy for every training participant by visiting http://www.balboapress.com.au.

The Ride of Your Life Workbook

About this Workbook

This workbook is a guide to understanding yourself as a human being. It focuses on how to run your life.

The exercises look at what you do and why you do it. Completing them permits you to uncover who you currently think you are. It helps you look at influences from your past and create a future of your choice.

How to Use This Workbook

There is no right or wrong way to use this workbook. However, I do suggest that you keep a pencil in hand to jot down personal thoughts you may have along the way.

You can use this workbook individually or in small groups. When used as a group workbook, the exchange of experiences between participants usually gives rise to human insights that you could never find on your own.

Even after you read this workbook, it can continue to serve as a reference guide. Like any journey, repeated visits will invariably lead to elements overlooked previously.

This is a personal journey of discovery. Encourage and permit yourself to make personal notes. It is through self-reflection that you may learn who you are. This is the ride of your life.

Exercise 1: To Start

Draw a horse-drawn carriage.

- 1 horse (pulling a carriage)
- 1 driver (sitting in the driver's seat, holding the reins)
- 1 master (inside the carriage)
- Place the carriage on a road.

The Ride of Your Life Model

The Ride of Your Life model comes to us from ancient oriental writings in which a person's life is compared to a ride in a horse-drawn carriage. The carriage represents the physical body; the horse represents the emotions; the driver represents the mental faculties; and the person inside represents the inner self, who has chosen the road the carriage is to travel on. As a whole, this image represents our life's journey.

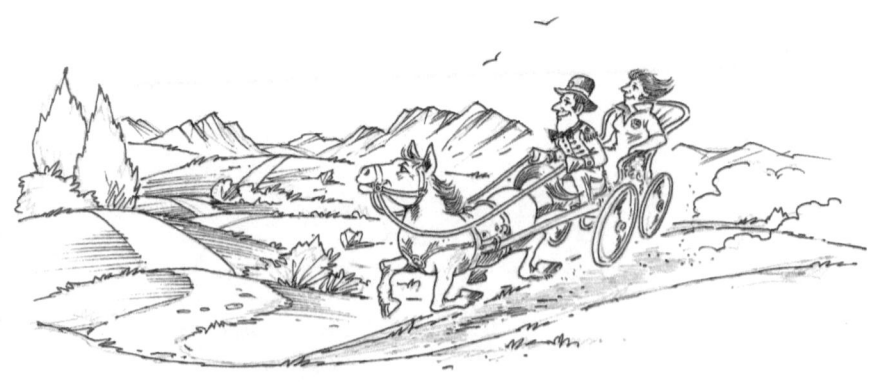

The Ride of Your Life Model Description

The carriage	=	The physical body
A horse pulling a carriage	=	The emotions
A driver steering the carriage	=	The thoughts
A master inside the carriage	=	The inner self
The road	=	The journey of life

The purpose of the Ride of Your Life model is to gain mastery to run your own life. Mastery is obtained when all your parts—carriage, horse, driver, and master—work together.

Look at the picture you drew, and compare it to what you now know about the model. From this picture, can you obtain clues or insights into the way you experience yourself?

> ❖ *My husband drew a very royal-looking horse, driver, and an open carriage with a queen sitting inside. I thought this revealed his feminine side.*
>
> ❖ *My daughter Danielle drew a cuddly teddy bear rather than a horse pulling her carriage. She was a teenager at this time and noted that sometimes her teddy bear turned into a grizzly bear.*

For the sake of understanding the Ride of Your Life model, the next five chapters of this workbook look at each separate component carefully.

Carriage	=	Physical
Horse	=	Emotional
Driver	=	Mental
Master	=	Inner self
Road	=	Life's adventure

The Carriage

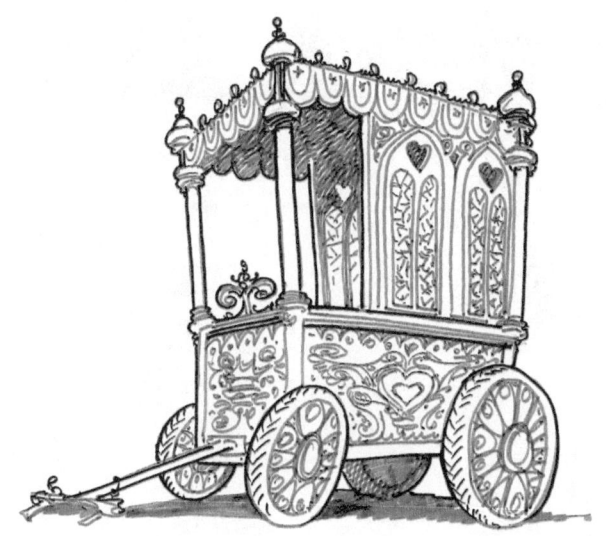

Jacquie Robinson

The Carriage = the Physical Body

The specific properties—colour, shape, and characteristics—of your carriage came from your ancestors.

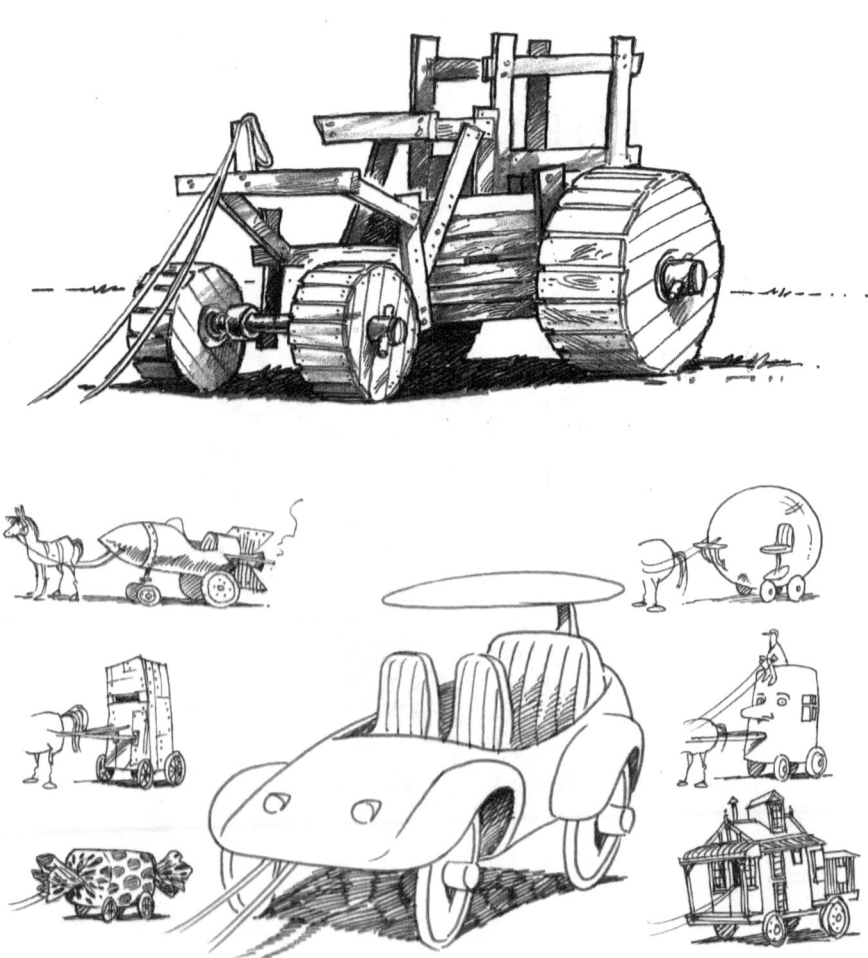

EXERCISE 2: FAMILY TREE

Fill in your family tree below. Think about the physical features of your carriage as they were passed down to you from generation to generation.

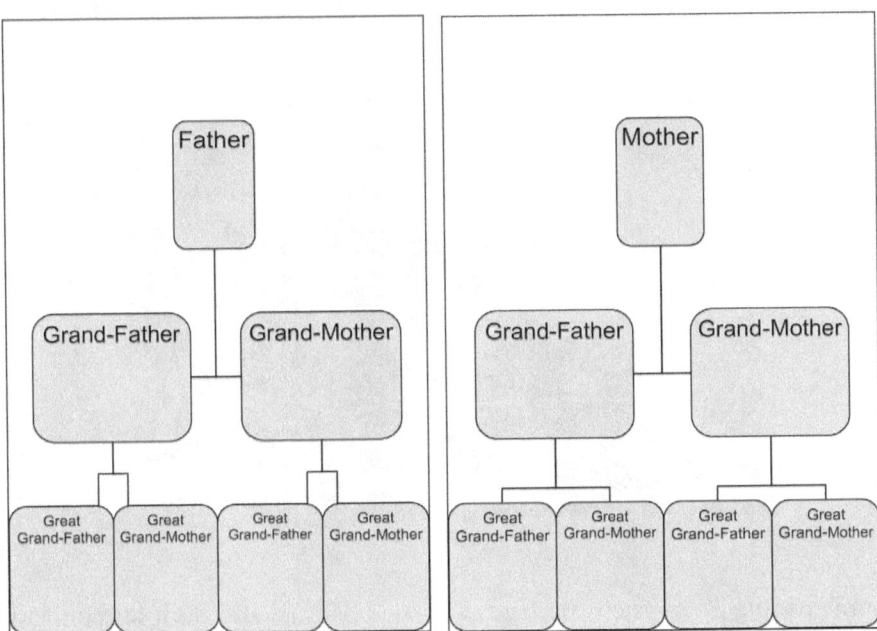

Although the colour of your skin, your build, and the shape of your body resemble others in your family, this does not mean that you have no choice with respect to your carriage's appearance. Think about how you are physically. Are you in good physical shape? Do you keep your body clean? Do you exercise regularly? Do you eat healthy food?

If well cared for, our carriages (bodies) will last for many years. If treated carelessly, they tend to break down and wear out—and replacement parts may not be readily available.

In your infancy, your parents cared for your carriage. As you grew and became more coordinated, you were gradually given the responsibility of caring for it yourself. As an adult, if you do not take care of your body, nobody else will; full responsibility for the care and maintenance of your carriage is yours alone.

A carriage that is unclean and uncared for may provide a very unpleasant ride.

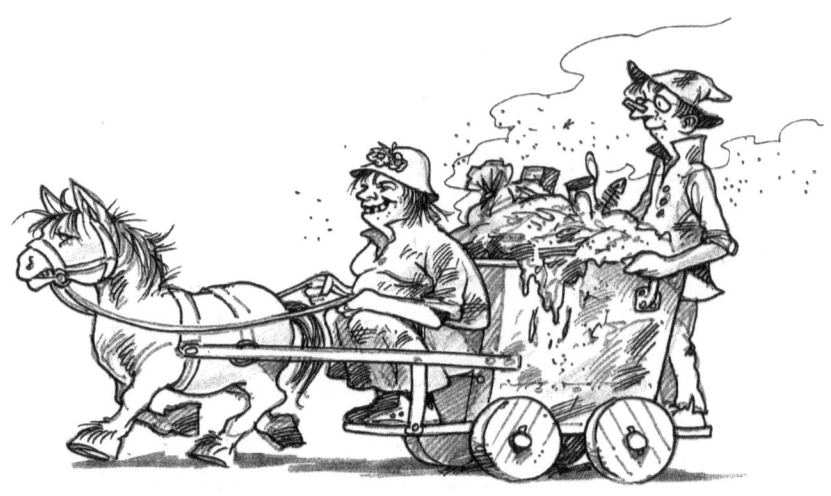

Some people prefer their carriage to be well padded and built for comfort rather than speed.

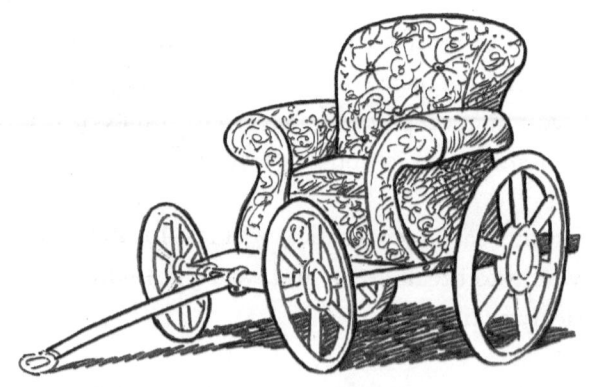

The Carriage Ride

Others choose to keep their carriage sleek, well oiled, and streamlined.

Some people think of their carriage as simply a means to get around.

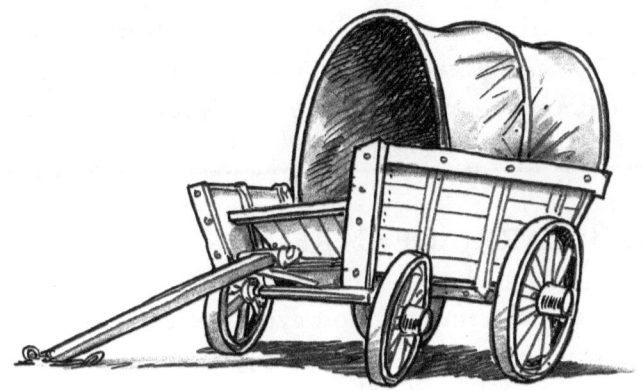

> *My husband and I had a pleasant surprise recently when we used a physical-assessment machine at our local gym. (We make a point of going to the gym twice a week.) At the time of writing this, my husband's actual age is sixty-six, but his metabolic age according to the machine is that of a man of thirty-five. I am fifty-five, and my metabolic age is that of a woman eleven years younger. I told my husband that he would have to learn to respect his elders. His quick reply was to say that he would need to tell everyone that he is now married to an older woman.*

EXERCISE 3: CARRIAGE CARE

There are professional trainers at most gyms who can give you a physical-fitness assessment and provide a personal programme to fit your needs. Many gyms have a machine that looks like a simple bathroom scale, but instead of only telling you your weight, it gives your percentage of body fat (both visceral and external), your bone density, and your metabolic age. Make a point of going to your gym to discover how fit you are. Take care of your carriage; it has to last you a lifetime!

Exercise 4: Physical Fitness

Take a moment and think about your carriage as it is now. Write brief statements about the following.

What aches and pains do you have?
_____
_____

How easily do you move?
_____
_____

Are you carrying extra weight?
_____
_____

Are you in desperate need of some repairs?
_____
_____

What is your plan to take care of your carriage?
_____
_____

Jacquie Robinson

EXERCISE 5: HORSE-DRAWN CARRIAGES

Below is a list of horse-drawn carriages. Circle the one that best describes how you currently see your physical body.

> Ambulance
> Armoured vehicle
> Beer wagon
> Buggy (open)
> Buggy (closed)
> Carnival wagon
> Chariot
> Cinderella's pumpkin coach
> Dogcatcher's wagon
> Firetruck
> Garbage wagon
> Hackney carriage
> Hearse
> Ice wagon
> Manure spreader
> Maple-sugar sled
> Medicine wagon
> Milk wagon
> Pastry or bakery wagon
> Prince Charming's royal coach
> Prison wagon
> Racing cart
> Royal coach
> Show carriage
> Sleigh
> Stagecoach
> Sulky racer
> Wine-barrel wagon

Now, put a smiley face beside which kind of carriage you would like to have in the future, the one you are motivated to work towards obtaining.

The Carriage Ride

Remember to take care of your carriage.
There is a special passenger inside:
YOU!

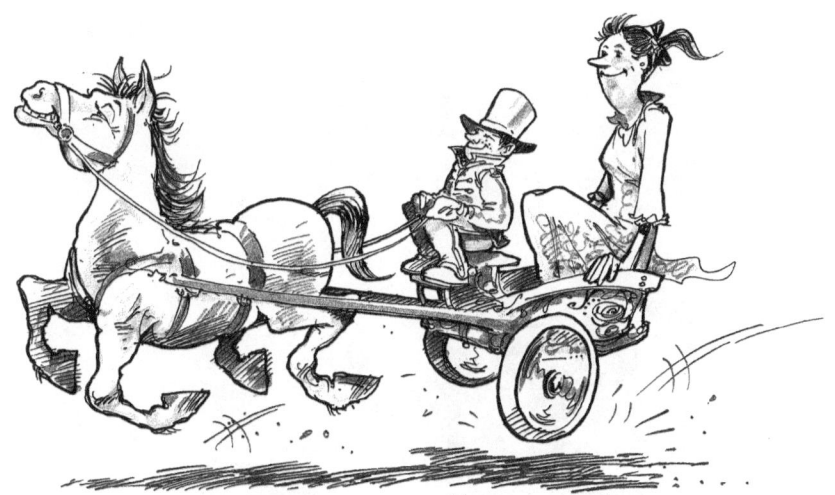

The Horse

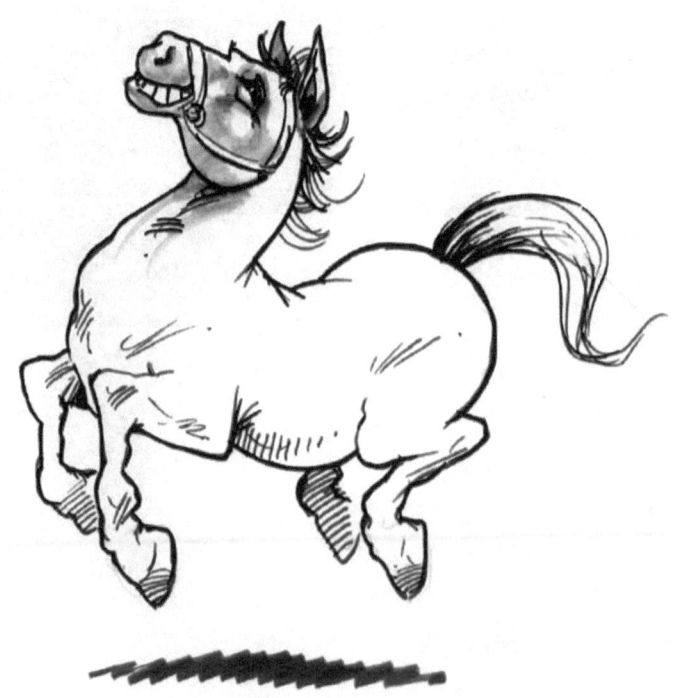

THE HORSE = EMOTIONS

Your emotions are the horse that pulls your carriage.

Like the horse that provides the energy for the carriage to move, your emotions provide the energy you need to move along in life. When you are happy, you have an abundance of energy. When you are sad, simply getting out of bed in the morning may become very difficult. When you are depressed or upset, going anywhere or doing anything may become just plain hard work.

Your emotions are innately primitive and natural. When something frightens you, you jump. When you feel threatened, you run away, prepare to fight, or freeze in your tracks. This is how you and the rest of the animal world are programmed. Flight, fight, or freeze are natural, instinctive, and emotional reactions.

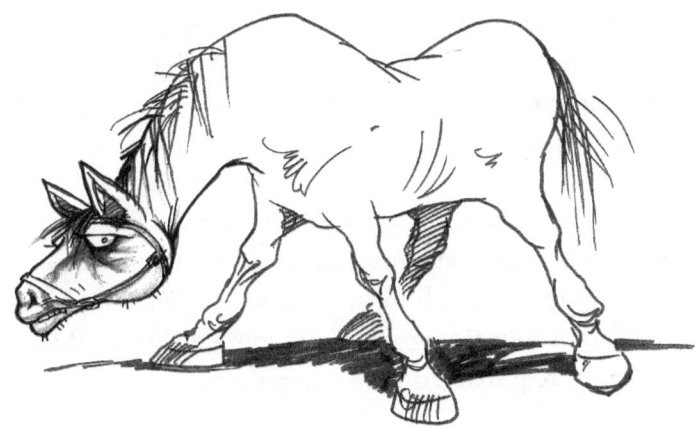

I grew up around horses and other farm animals. My grandfather had a team of huge draught workhorses. My uncles used quarter horses to round up their beef cattle and bred thoroughbred racehorses that were renowned for their speed. How different these horses are from each other!

The workhorses were gentle giants, calm and easily handled. They permitted us to jump on and off their bare backs without taking any notice of us while Grandpa led them around the farmyard.

Jacquie Robinson

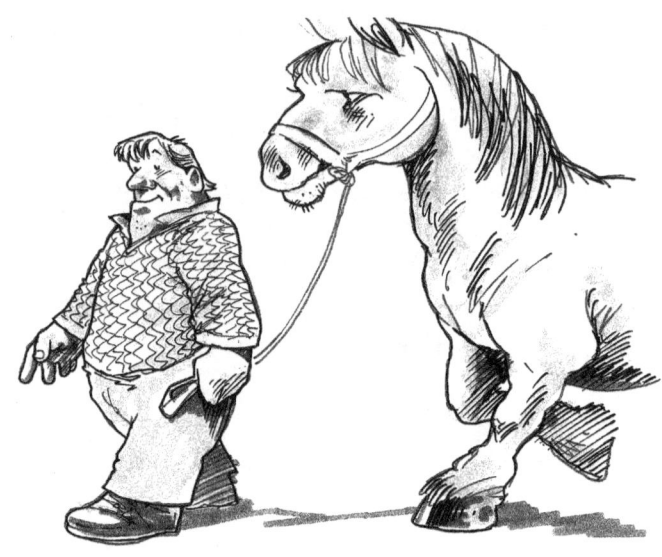

The quarter horses were swift and agile and loved to gallop. We rode them with cowboy saddles that had a large pummel. We hung on to this tightly as these horses could turn sharply, leaving us facing in one direction while they headed off in another.

The thoroughbred racehorses were built for speed. They were excitable, extremely alert, and highly athletic creatures. We were not permitted to ride them; they were too much for us to manage. We could brush them and clean their stalls, but riding them was completely forbidden. Each of the different horses required a different approach.

Draught workhorses are known to be calm and easy-going, while thoroughbreds are considered to be extremely alert and highly athletic. As individual humans, however, we each have an emotional disposition that is an acquired, habitual nature composed of a combination of our emotions and behaviours.

The Carriage Ride

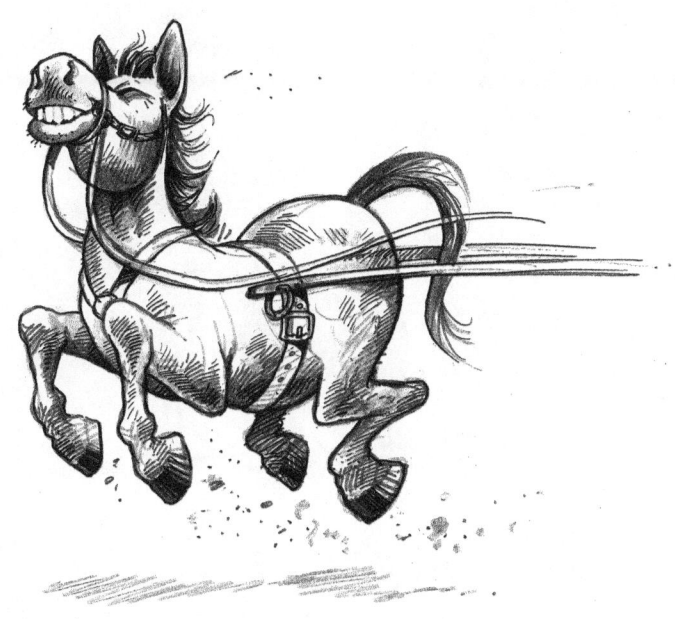

Some people are very emotional, easily excitable, and highly responsive. Others can be angry, aggressive, fierce, even irritable, seeming more like a grizzly bear than a person. I have also met people who are shy, fearful, and extremely anxious; they remind me of frightened rabbits. Emotions can set you in motion or stop you in your tracks. Is it any wonder that learning how to control your horse (your emotions) instead of letting it (them) run away with you is a lifelong challenge? Are you able to bridle your emotions—or do they run your life? How do you use this energy to take you down the road you want to travel? Do you run your emotions, or do they run you?

Jacquie Robinson

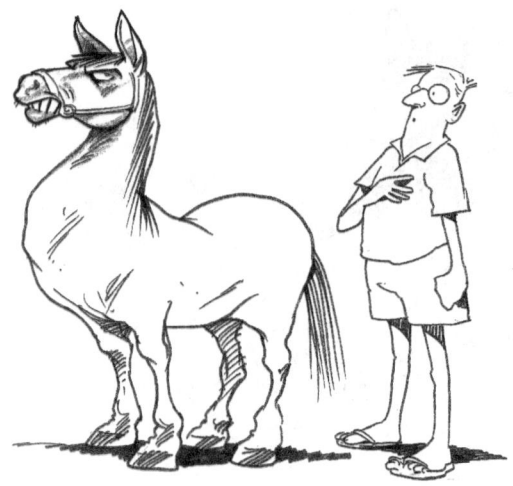

How would you best describe your horse (your emotions)?

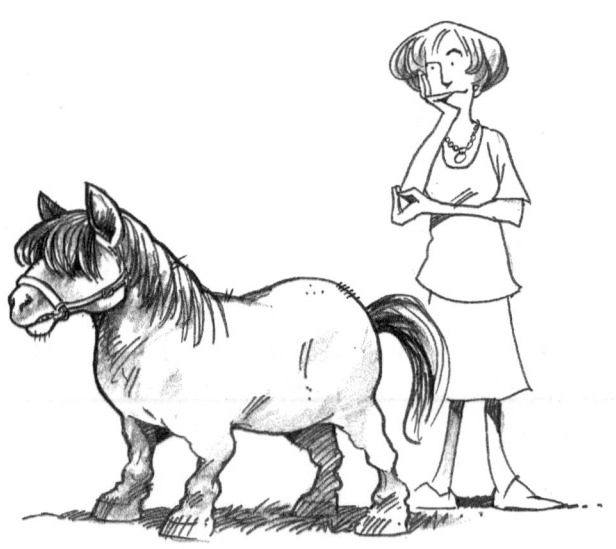

EXERCISE 6: HORSE BREEDS

There are many breeds of horses, each with their own dispositions. For this next exercise, I would like you to research the characteristics of each breed; this information is readily available online. Once you have had a chance to peruse the various breed-specific characteristics, select the breed that most resembles your disposition.

Next, ask your friends to select the breed they think most accurately reflects you.

You may be surprised at how others perceive you compared to how you perceive yourself.

Here are some examples of emotions (in alphabetical order) that you may relate to. Circle the ones you feel at the moment, and put a smiley face on the ones that you would like to nourish in the future.

List of Emotions

How are you feeling at this moment?

Abandoned	Closed	Disgusted
Abused	Closed off	Dishonest
Accused	Clumsy	Dismissed
Affected	Complex	Disorganised
Aggressed	Condescended	Disoriented
Aggressive	Condoned	Disputed
Ambivalent	Confounded	Dissatisfied
Angry	Confused	Distrustful
Annoyed	Contained	Dominant
Anxious	Coward	Dominated
Arrogant	Demanding	Embarrassed
Astonished	Demolished	Enraged
Attacked	Dependent	Envious
Betrayed	Depressed	Excluded
Blame	Destroyed	Furious
Censored	Disappointed	Grouchy

Guilty	Judged	Shameful
Hesitant	Left out	Shocked
Hostile	Malicious	Shoved
Humiliating	Manipulated	Shy
Hurt	Melancholic	Stubborn
Idiot	Mischievous	Stunned
Ill-treated	Miserable	Subjugated
Inadequate	Misunderstood	Submissive
Incapable	Monitored	Surpassed
Incensed	Not respected	Torn
Indifferent	Off Perplexed	Touched
Infantile	Persecuted	Unhappy
Innocent	Proud	Unjust
Insensitive	Remote	Unreasonable
Insulted	Reprimanded	Unworthy
Intimidated	Ridiculed	Used
Intolerant	Rigid	Worried
Invaded	Sad	Wronged
Isolated	Sarcastic	Wrongful
Jealous	Scared	

The Driver

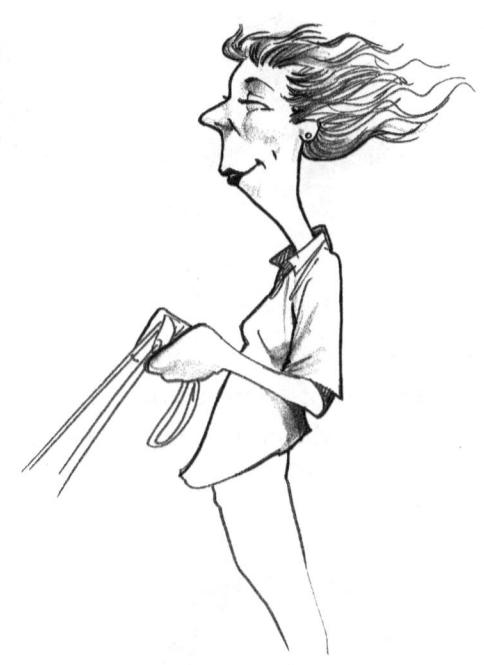

THE DRIVER = YOUR THINKING

The driver represents the way you think.

The driver of your carriage has control of your horse (your emotions). Your horse provides your energy, but your driver holds the reins. Discovering how to drive or control your emotions is a lifelong learning experience.

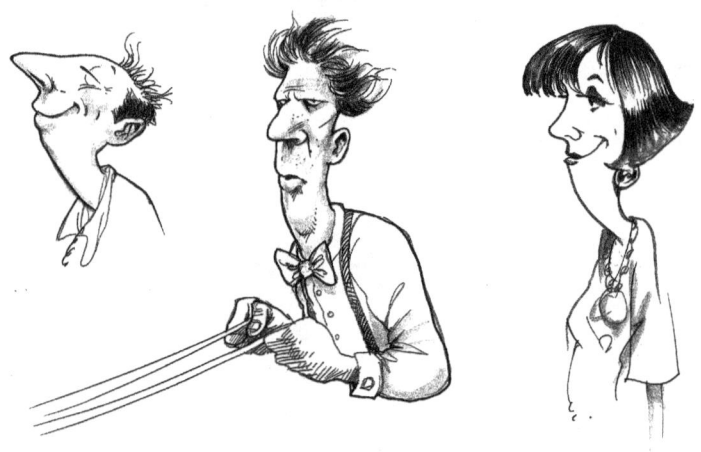

Think back to when you were a young child. Do you remember times when your emotions got out of control, when your happiness, anger, sadness, and/or fear were overwhelming? Have you ever thought, *I wish I could just feel happy*?

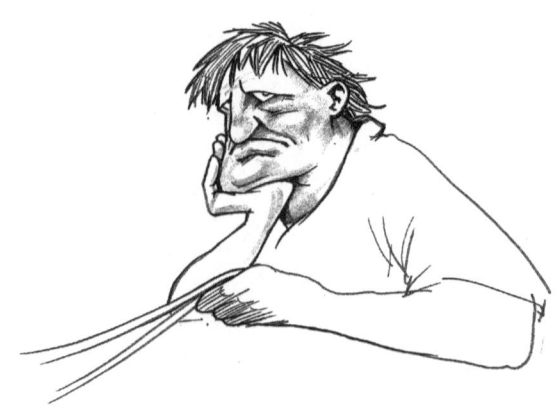

The Carriage Ride

Do you remember ever blaming others for your emotions? Do you remember ever making the following comments: "You made me angry," "You hurt my feelings," "You made me sad," or, "You frightened me."? Then, after these statements, do you remember expecting the other person to do or say something to make you feel better?

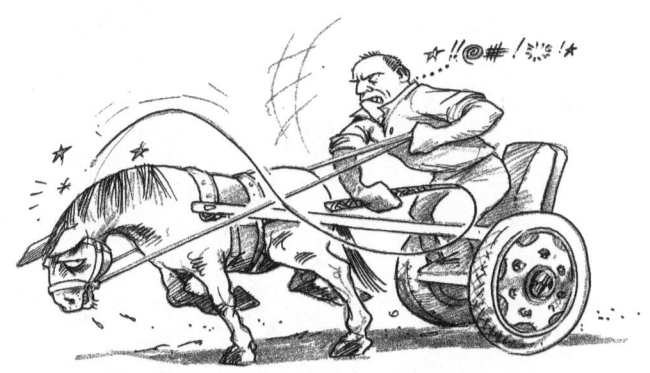

Do you ever tell yourself, "I'm not good enough," or "smart enough"? Do you ever hear yourself getting impatient and saying, "Hurry up!" "You're going too slowly," "You're taking too long," "You should be faster, better, quicker," and things like that? Such thinking is like driving your horse with a whip.

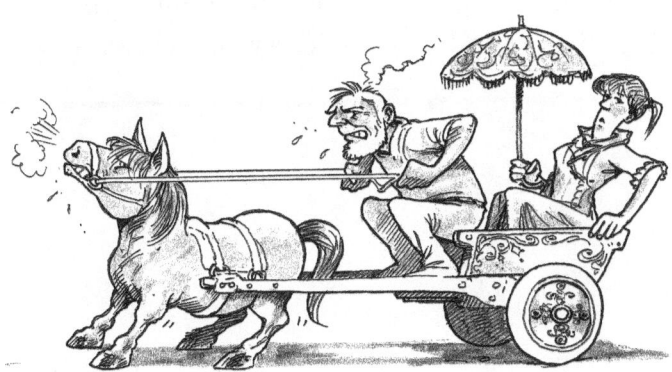

Angry and frustrated thinking makes a frustrated, upset horse and a captive passenger.

Jacquie Robinson

Exercise 7: You Make Me Feel

The driver controls the horse with the tightness of the reins and uses his or her voice to talk to the horse, slowing and calming it down or encouraging it to go faster. This is the same way your thoughts affect your emotions. You can think of any situation as fun, a great adventure, stressful, undesirable, or as hard work.

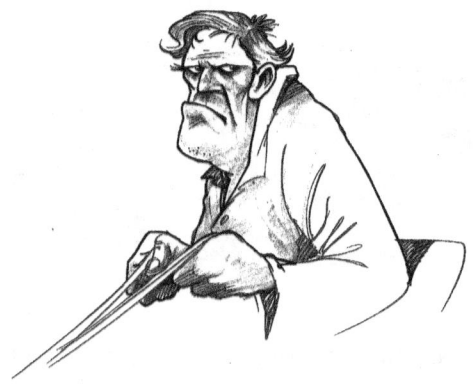

In the box provided, make a note or draw a picture of how you drive your horse. A good time to become aware of your driver is first thing in the morning when you get out of bed. If you are still not certain, during the next part of your day, note how you talk to yourself in any given situation.

The Carriage Ride

A Note to "Drunk Drivers"

You can lose control of your emotions if you choose to drink and drive. This leaves your horse (emotions) in control rather than your driver.

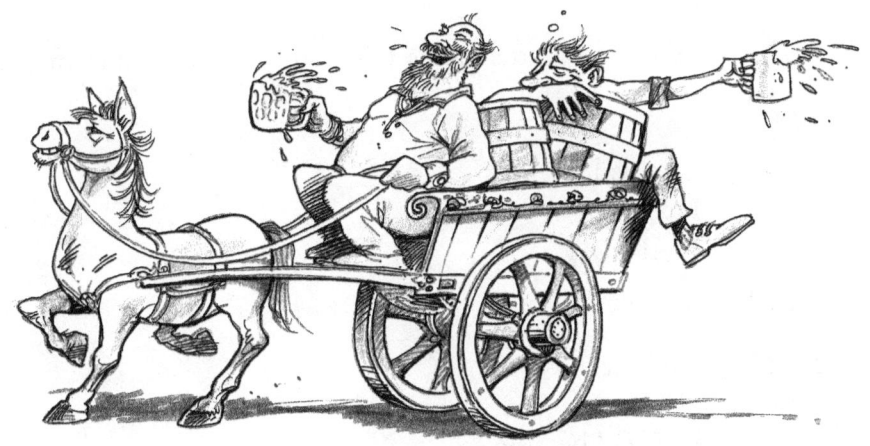

Exercise 8: Distinguish Your Thoughts from Your Feelings

The Ride of Your Life model allows you to distinguish your thoughts from your feelings.

1. Notice the *thoughts* that come into your mind the moment you say the following.

    a. "I feel sad."
    b. "I feel happy."
    c. "I feel angry."
    d. "I feel jealous."

2. Then add "because."

    a. "I feel sad because ..."
    b. "I feel happy because ..."
    c. "I feel angry because ..."
    d. "I feel jealous because ..."

3. The "because" is the entity that you are holding responsible for your feelings; the "cause" of the matter. Your emotions respond to what you think. You are not troubled by what happens to you; you are troubled by your thoughts regarding what happens.

Permit me to tell you one of my aunt Nonie's stories to help you understand this concept.

> We had two water wells; one at the house, and the other back at the bush. Somebody had to walk back to the bush well and pump water for the cattle. Mostly, this was done in the evening, just before dark. One evening it was my job to pump water, which went into a water trough. We were supposed to leave it full after the cattle had finished drinking, but it was getting dark before I had the tank full. I noticed some bright lights in the grass. I was sure they were the eyes of

some wild animal with sharp teeth and long claws, sneaking out of the bush to eat little girls. Oh, I was scared. I ran as fast as I could. I ran straight to the safety of the house. Every time I looked back, the eyes seemed to be getting closer. When I reached the house, out of breath, I was told it was not wild animals at all, just fireflies in their mating season.

Many years later, my little son, Bryce, saw the same phenomenon and rushed into the house all excited to tell me he saw the "fairies" lighting their lights and asked if he could he go and play with them.

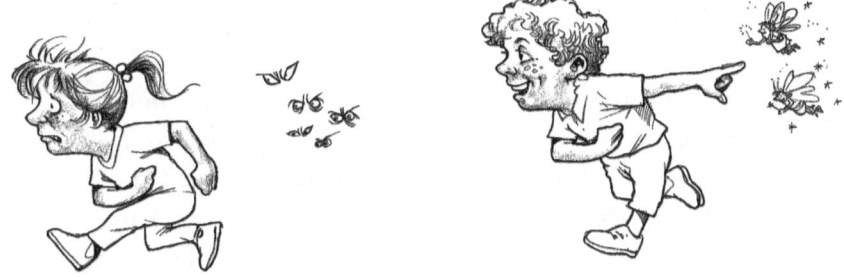

Aunt Nonie thought *wild animals* when she saw the fireflies. This thought suggested danger and made her feel afraid. Bryce thought *fairies*. This thought painted a picture in his mind of fun and made him feel happy, wanting to go and play. Emotions certainly do respond to thoughts.

I had an experience when I was a little girl staying overnight at my favourite aunt's place (Aunt Nonie, of course).

> It was bedtime, and I was to sleep in the front porch bedroom. After reading me a story and kissing me goodnight, she left, turning off the light. There, suddenly at the door, appeared a huge monster. I screamed in terror. Aunt Nonie quickly returned. When she opened the door and turned on the lights, I was certain the monster had hid behind the door. She looked, but it was not there anymore. I was certain that it was hiding somewhere and

did not want her to leave me alone. I told her that there was a big, huge "monster" that was going to get me. She gave me a hug, calmed me down, and said that she would stay with me when she turned the lights off again to see if the monster would dare to come back out with her there. It did. As soon as she turned the lights out, the big monster appeared suddenly as it had before. Aunt Nonie fearlessly got up and took a step towards it, stepping between the monster and the porch window. It disappeared magically, and I cheered and clapped because it was afraid of her. However, when she came back to sit with me, it jumped out of the dark again. I screamed for her to turn around quickly, so she could see.

Aunt Nonie calmly explained to me that the monster was the reflection of the bedpost onto the door from the moonlight coming in the porch windows, and I didn't need to be afraid. Together we made the monster shadow disappear by taking away its light. I did it several times on my own and felt very brave, no longer afraid. I thought, *I am very strong, stronger than the shadow monster because I can take away its light and make it disappear.*

Aunt Nonie's story and my own experience led me to begin taking note of my thoughts, testing out their validity, and watching how my thinking could directly influence my emotions. I was beginning to understand how to drive my horse.

Learning to Drive Your Horse (Emotions)

Thinking and expressing emotions is part of what makes us human. Many people, however, when children were encouraged not to show their emotions and made to believe that expressing them was a sign of weakness. Consequently, many people become disconnected to their emotions and are unable to manage them.

The Carriage Ride

Most of us learn to drive our emotions by trial and error. You are given brief instructions, and more often than not, there are essential details missing. You usually learn after the fact; when you are brought up short with some type of scolding or are disciplined with some type of time out—or something harsher. This happens when letting your emotions run you has led you into a potential dangerous situation. Steering your emotions, like riding a horse or driving a car, requires full control.

Let me tell you the story of my aunt Nonie's learning to drive a car to illustrate. My Aunt Nonie had always in the past either hitched up the horse and buggy to go somewhere or simply walked if it was close enough. This was until my Uncle Harvey bought their first car. When they got it home, my Uncle Harvey bet her that she could not drive it to the corner and back. He showed her how it worked: the gas pedal to go, the brake pedal to stop, put it in drive to go forward, and reverse to back up.

Aunt Nonie got in, put the car in drive, stepped on the gas pedal, and drove to the corner. Once there, she stomped her foot on the brake and stopped. She then put the car in reverse, stepped on the gas pedal, and drove backwards all the way back home. She took her foot off the gas and stomped on the brake. She had made it to the corner, back, and won her bet. She said, "Now I can drive!" (Although she did not know that you used the brake to slow down. She thought it was only used to stop. She figured you just took your foot off the gas pedal a lot or a bit to go slower.)

The next day she decided she would drive to see her neighbour who lived on the next farm up the hill instead of walking as she usually did. Getting there was no problem. She just repeated the way she had driven to the corner. Getting back, however, was more difficult. Uncle Harvey yesterday had scolded her for driving so far and so fast backwards on the road. Therefore, when she was to leave, she drove around the neighbour's house to get back on the road to head downhill towards home. As she got closer, she took her foot off the gas pedal, expecting to slow down. However, the car did not slow down. In fact, it gathered speed. She knew the car was going very fast, and she was not sure how she was going to turn into their laneway. Therefore, she just whipped it in and stomped on the brake, coming to a skidding stop right in front of her house. She was glad to be home safe and quite pleased with herself.

Uncle Harvey came running out of the house and told her that he had seen daylight under the wheels when she made the turn. What was she thinking to try to turn when going so fast? He told her next time to use the brake to slow down before attempting any turning. *Well,* she thought, *now I know how to go, how to stop, and how to slow down. I am ready now to take my driver's test.*

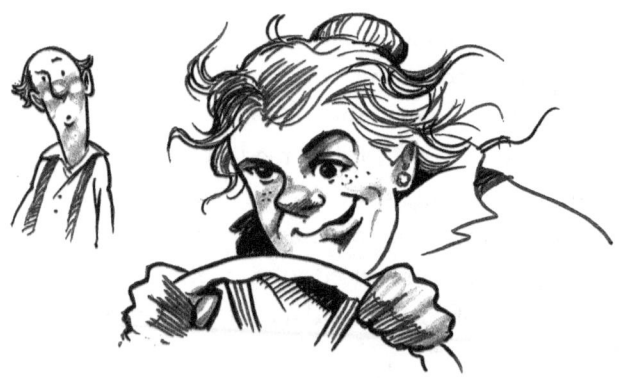

She drove the next day to Seaforth to take her test. The driving examiner was not too pleased that she had driven herself there; didn't she know you needed a license to drive? *What a silly question,* she thought. Of course she did. That was why she was there. So they started the driver's test being cross with each other. She came to a corner at the highway, she recounts, and he told her to turn right, so she did. He yelled at her, "Don't you know enough to stop before turning onto the highway?"

Aunt Nonie, ready to give as good as she got, responded, "When they want me to stop, they will put up a stop sign." You know something? She told us right after she got her driver's license, stop signs sprouted up all over the place around Cromarty, where she lived.

Uncle Harvey was certain the examiner gave her the license because he had escaped with his life and was not going to take another chance with her taking the test again as he may not be so lucky a second time. Better safe than sorry.

As you can see, driving a car requires full instructions and guidance to permit clear understanding and promote the required skills—just like learning how to drive your emotions. You often learn from trial and error, just the way Aunt Nonie did. What you also do from the beginning of your life in order to learn is watch the people around you and take on or reject their examples. Take, for example, your family. You have observed your parents, grandparents, uncles, aunts, cousins, brothers, sisters, and others express and receive love and affection as well as demonstrate anger and sadness. They set an example for you to follow. Just possibly the way you express your emotions is very similar to your family members' whether you are aware of it or not.

According to Eric Bern's Transactional Analysis, there are five conditional "drivers" or ways you can think that will cause you to live your life to please others. They are:

1. Be strong.
2. Be perfect.
3. Try harder.
4. Hurry up.
5. Be unselfish.

Jacquie Robinson

Do you drive yourself with any of Bern's conditional drivers?

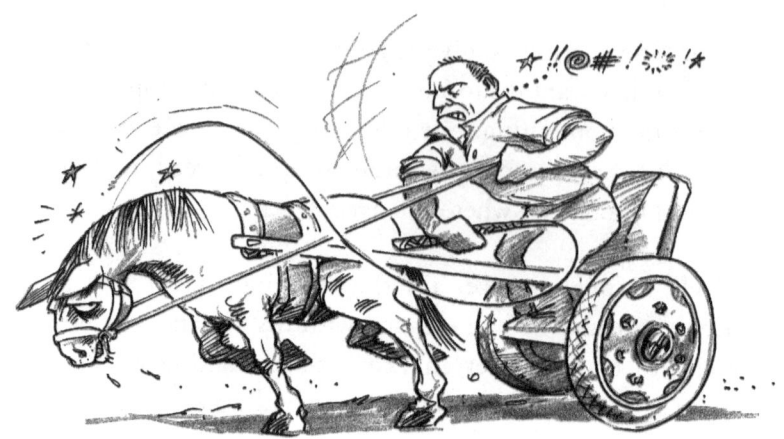

EXERCISE 9: LIFE IS NOT FAIR

When you think that "life should be fairer," you experience one of the six emotions or feelings that can make you miserable. Is this the ride of your life?

F	Fear
A	Anger
I	Insecurity
R	Regret
E	Envy
R	Resentment

Live Your Life Creatively

According to Roger Van Oech, the author of the 'Creative Whack Pack', a deck of 84 thinking strategy cards, there are four types of thinking that can help you live your life creatively. You can think like an:

1) Explorer—Focusing on discovering resources to create new ideas.
2) Artist—Focusing on transforming resources into something creative.
3) Judge—Focusing on evaluating ideas as to their value and or merit.
4) Warrior—Focusing on implementing the ideas.

Jacquie Robinson

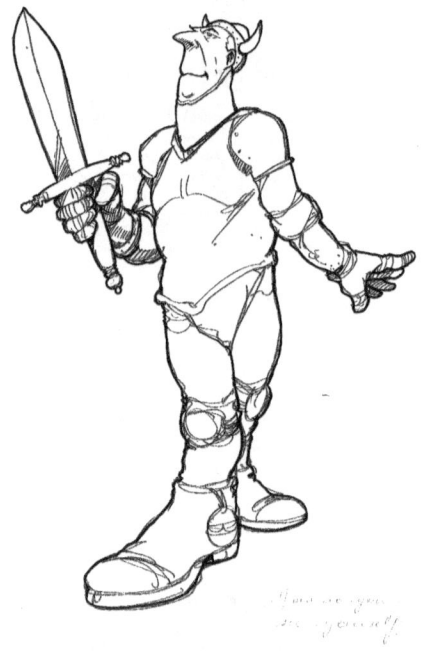

Van Oech Creative Whack Pack of cards are fun to use to help learn how to think creatively. I often pick a card when my mind has begun to drive me around and around in circles. The Whack Pack also now is an app.

The Carriage Ride

Self-Talk

Discovering the right words to say and use is important for drivers. Think of a coachman without the words for start or stop. What you tell yourself can be motivating, encouraging, calming, and so on, all the way along a scale from positive to the most negative, where you are mentally beating your poor horse into the ground.

If you have ever had the opportunity to drive a real horse, you will understand the importance of knowing how to handle and control your animal. A fearful, inexperienced driver has little chance of getting the horse to go where he or she wants it to go.

The best jockeys who drive horses for a living have received years of instruction, guidance, and hands-on experience. They have learnt how to encourage their mounts to give their best. Learning to drive your horse requires nothing less. You need to know how to get the best from yourself.

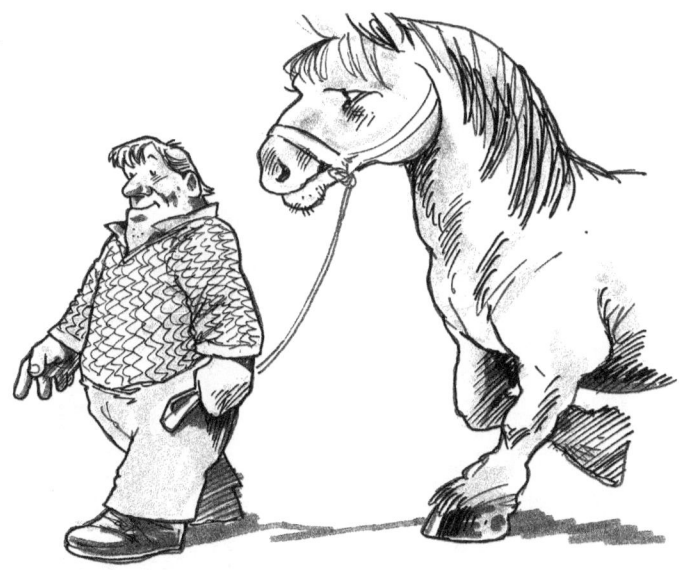

Think over and listen to how you talk to yourself. Observe what you say and how you interact. Your thoughts can direct you eagerly forward, seeking adventure and fun. Or they can just as easily imagine problems or difficulties, directing your horse/emotions to be overly cautious and anxious. These are just two possibilities. There are many thoughts that directly influence our emotional states.

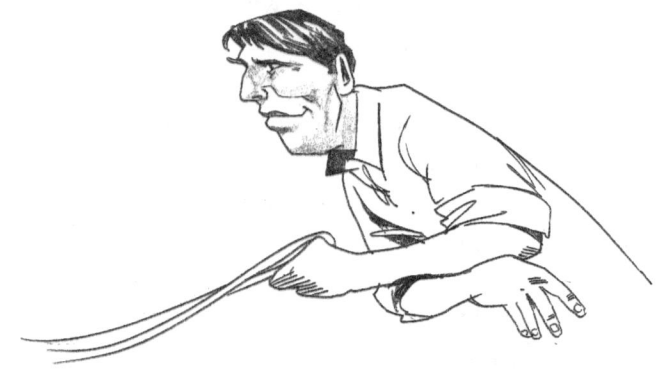

Exercise 10: Self-Talk

Listen to your thoughts in the situations you encounter. Note the feelings that are evoked.

The Event	Your Self-Talk	Your Feelings

··· ··· ···

The Master—The Inner Self

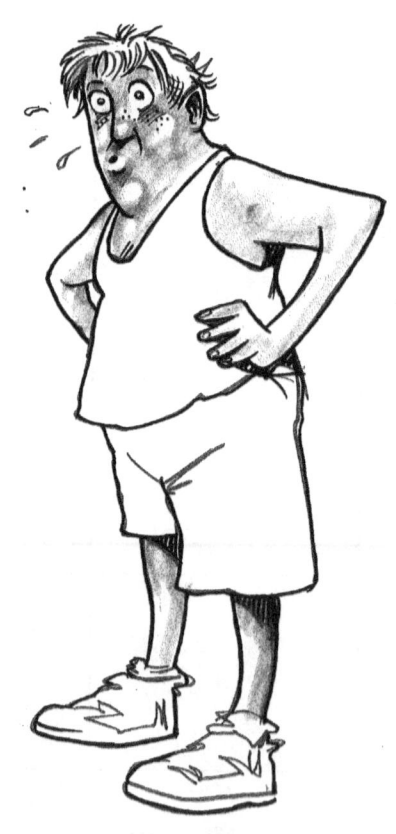

THE MASTER—THE INNER SELF

The master represents your inner self. Some people may prefer to think of the inner self as your soul or spiritual self. Whichever word you use, it is your master inside the carriage who is responsible for choosing the image of how you see yourself and, ultimately, the Ride of Your Life.

When you take a taxi ride, you get to tell the driver where you want to go. If you have not chosen a specific destination, how can you expect the driver to take you anywhere? In the ride of your life, if your master can give specific directions to your driver as to your desired destination, there is a possibility to advance to that place. Otherwise, there is no possibility at all.

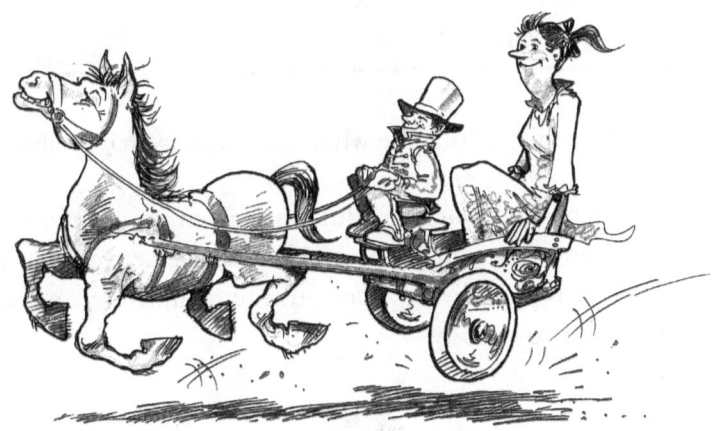

Within you is the ability, possibility and power to be whatever you want to be and go wherever you want to go. Do what it takes to make yourself a success and happy. More often than not, when you haven't chosen where you want to go or when you believe that you can't get there, it's impossible, the driver returns to old, familiar roads. You end up repeating your past or wandering through life lost and wishing things were different, believing that things will never change ... unless?

Learning how to define what you really want, to make clear goals, and to set a course you wish to take are the keys to success. Whichever direction your master chooses your driver will take as a command. What you, the master inside your carriage, holds out as a possible future destination for you is where you ultimately end up.

I have overheard people give the following directions to their drivers.

> - "My life is always an uphill journey; nothing is ever easy."
> - "Things always go wrong in my life no matter what I try to do."
> - "I'll never be able to do anything in my life."
> - "I'm not good enough or smart enough to get ahead in life."
> - "I don't know what I want. I don't really want anything from life."
> - "Everything's just too hard in my life."
> - "What a rotten, miserable life I have."
> - "I don't deserve to be happy."

With these beliefs, can you imagine what destinations are possible?

If your master has no hope for the future, has given up on life, does not care what you do or where you go, and feels dead inside, you are driving a hearse. You have stopped living, shut out life completely, and are just waiting to dispose of your body.

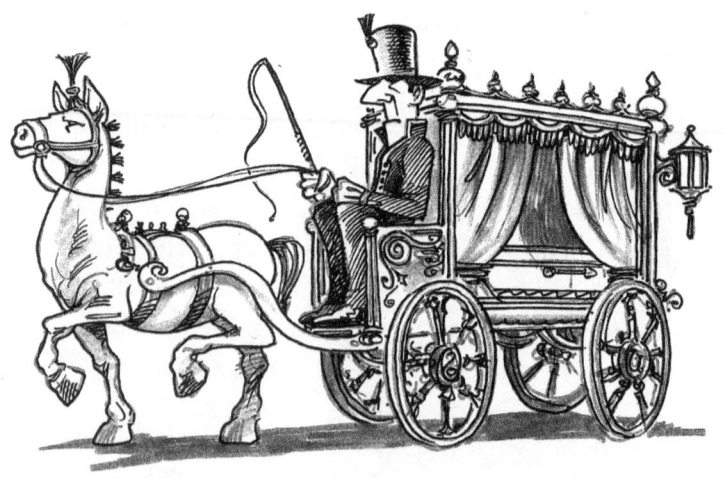

Inner Beliefs

Have you ever considered how much of what you do, how you act, and how successful you are is dependent on your beliefs about yourself? Your values matter as they define the way you live your life.

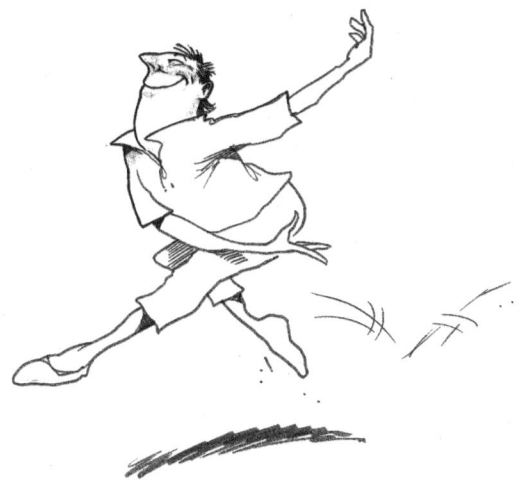

Imagine what you would do differently if you believed you were someone else, if you had a different past, or you were at a different place in your present life. Where would you go? What would you do with your new life? If you were free to choose what you wanted in your life, what would you want? If you were free to have the ride of your life, what life would you choose?

Your life depends on what you, the master inside your carriage, holds out as a possible future for you.

> My grandfather used to say:
>
> *"Reach for the moon for even if you miss, you will still end up among the stars."*

Exercise 11: Describing the Master

How would you describe your values, beliefs, and personal preferences?
How do you see yourself in your wildest possible dreams?
If anything were possible, what would you like to achieve in your life?

Circle the right answer for you.		
Are you masterful?	Yes	No
Do you want to go somewhere?	Yes	No
Do you know specifically where you want to go?	Yes	No
Are you content just where you are?	Yes	No
Are you looking for something interesting to do with your life?	Yes	No
Are you too absorbed in your own inner world to give any heed to where you want to go in your life?	Yes	No
Are you simply visiting, passing through this life to somewhere else?	Yes	No
Are you a spectator, an onlooker of what other people are doing in their lives and ignoring your own?	Yes	No
Does the life you are living feel like a prison sentence?	Yes	No

Are you enjoying your ride, watching and directing the trip?	Yes	No
Do you believe your life belongs to you?	Yes	No
Are you self-indulgent, excusing, and attribute responsibility of your life onto others?	Yes	No
Do you find that life is an adventure and look forward to the experience?	Yes	No

You are the master of the ride of your life. Your choice—your life. You are free to choose the ride of your life!

••• ••• •••

The Road

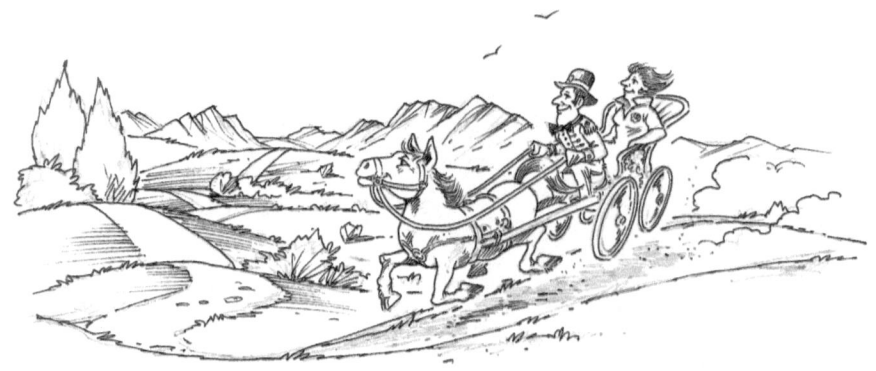

The Carriage Ride

THE ROAD = LIFE'S JOURNEY

The road represents your personal journey through life. The road is explored to establish your own existence and to fulfil your goals and capabilities. Your journey is the means whereby you discover and learn about who you are.

EXERCISE 12: DRAW A ROAD

In the box below, draw a road that climbs up a hill, descends into a valley, climbs up the other side, and goes straight again.

Mark the place on this road where you are now in your life, whether on top of a hill, way down in a valley, or somewhere in-between.

Jacquie Robinson

EXERCISE 13: PROBING YOUR LIFE'S JOURNEY

Write a description of your life's journey; a autobiography of sorts. Plot the most significant events in your life. This will help you to visualise the key features that have moved you along on your chosen path.

Recapture the unique, unrepeatable moments of your road. They are charged with personal events and stories. When revisited, they can give you a clearer picture of pieces of who you are and what has happened on your road.

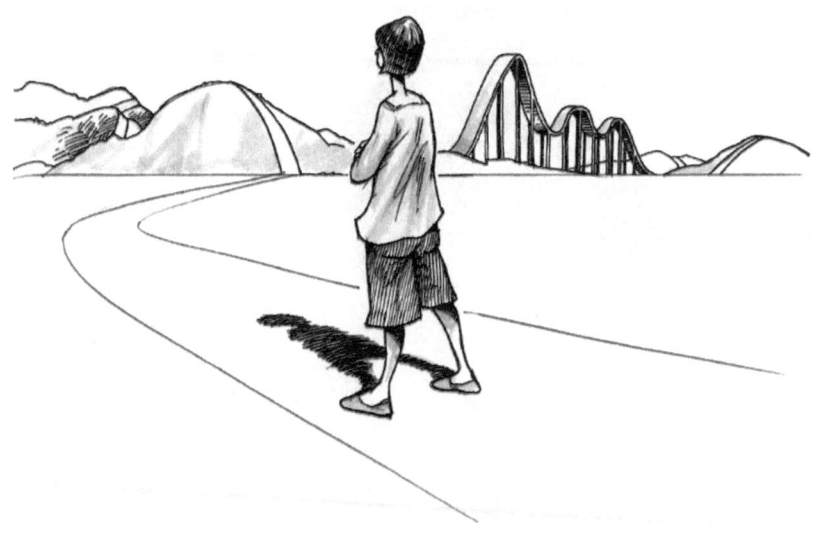

The Carriage Ride

EXERCISE 14: STORYBOARD

Storyboards are used to recall major events in your life. Name the events and then make an illustration to represent them in the squares provided. You then can plot these on your road map in the next exercise.

Major Life Event	Illustration

EXERCISE 15: DOT-TO-DOT ROAD MAP

Inside the circle below, place dots representing different events in your life. Label the dots. Think of them as places you have visited and explored, or stops you have made along your life's road. Join these dots together with lines representing a road from where you started in life to where you are now.

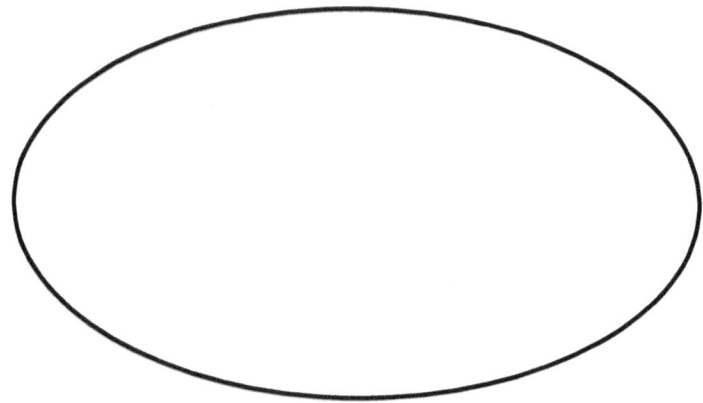

You can use this map to see where you have been and to help you plan where you would like to go. Place dots outside the circle indicating where you would like to see yourself five years from now along your road.

Memories form a complete record of your life, although you may not have conscious access to them. I think of them as reruns of movies that you can review. Knowing that they are available is important because you learn from them. Dwelling on the past can stop us from enjoying the present and having a future. Deciding to remain in the present is a personal choice.

Each place along your road has its links to your five senses (the three Ss and two Ts).

- Sight
- Sound
- Smell
- Taste
- Touch

Relive any of these senses, and you can return to the specific place in your life where you first experienced it. You can also use your five senses to bring you back to the present.

A great way to stop racing, anxious thoughts is to oblige yourself to look around where you are and find something orange. This is like the game of I spy with my little eye.

Exercise 16: The Three Ss and Two Ts

Identify the following.

- Five things you can see.
- Five things you can smell.
- Five sounds you can hear.
- Five things you can touch.
- Five things you can taste. (This one is optional as it may make you hungry.)

Personal Choice of How You See Your Road

Remember that where you have been does not dictate where you are going. The past does not equal the future. You may choose your future and change your road's direction at any time. It is a matter of personal choice. It is your life, open it up to possibilities, don't limit it to 'shoulds', 'if onlys', 'I can't', or 'mustn't'. How do you choose to experience your life's journey up to now? How do you imagine your future?

> *"The past existed in multitudinous ways. You only experienced one probable past. By changing this past in your mind now, in your present, you can change not only its nature but also its effect, and not only upon yourself but upon others."*
>
> *—Seth*

Blind Alleys, One-Way Streets, and Unexpected Events

Life does not always go as planned. Unexpected events happen. Life is an adventure, and if you try to avoid all surprises—if you attempt to control and plan everything—you shut out life and stop life itself.

The Carriage Ride

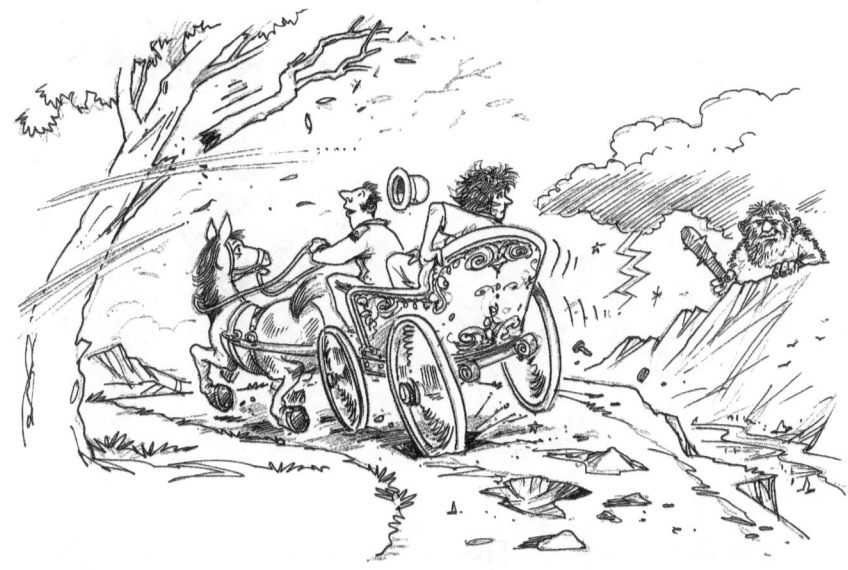

Most people keep their lives as constant as possible. (Change is scary!) However, this is like moving boringly along a straight, unremittingly flat road. Life truly lived has a closer resemblance to a roller-coaster ride.

I heard a tale that goes like this.

> One person says to the next, "I've had a perfect year."
> The other person naturally asks, "How did you manage that?"
> The first person replies, "Why, I was in a coma, of course."

Lives are not perfect; things happen. If you are living a perfect life, you are probably not doing anything new because it is almost impossible to attempt anything new without making mistakes. This is how you learn. When I was a child, my mother explained to me that I needed to make at least three mistakes a day. If I was not making mistakes, I was trying to be perfect, and I would then expect everyone around me to be perfect as well. She had met people who thought they were perfect, and they were not fun to be around at all. She hoped I would see life as a grand adventure and not be afraid to make mistakes. Being afraid to make mistakes, she said, stops people from ever trying anything new, doing anything, or going anywhere in their lives.

Jacquie Robinson

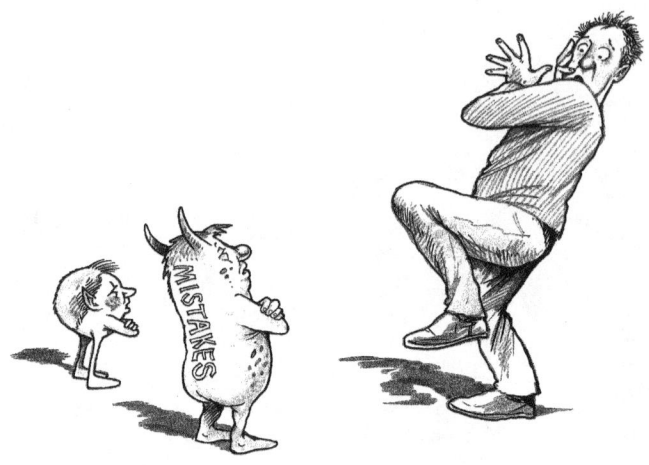

You can decide to give yourself permission to make at least three mistakes a day. I am certain you will find that doing so will give you the possibility of exploring life without fear of failure.

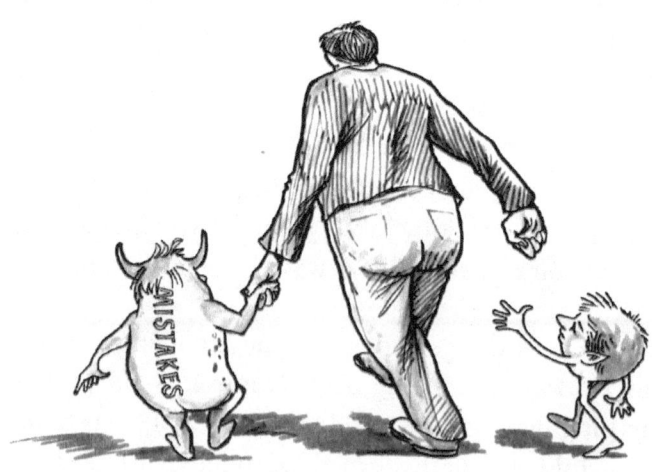

Your life's road does not have to be perfect, either. It does not have to turn out exactly as you planned. Everything and everyone does not have to behave in the way that you expect them to. People are not perfect, and neither are you.

The Carriage Ride

Starting out on a road that you have never explored before takes courage. You cannot guarantee what will happen.

By the very nature of exploring and adventuring, the results cannot be known in advance. Results emerge gradually from decisions and discoveries made along the way. The central idea of the Ride of Your Life model is to use your life's journey as an opportunity to learn and discover yourself.

> Life is an adventure.
> Life is a game
> Of follow the Road
> From where you came.
> Enjoy the present.
> Keep now in mind.
> Look ahead to the future
> And not behind.

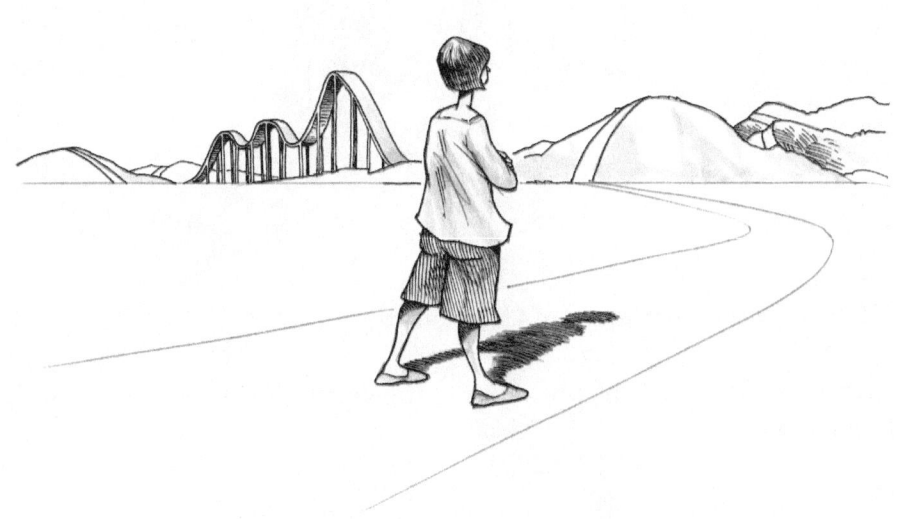

Jacquie Robinson

EXERCISE 17: OBSTACLES

Have there been obstacles that you have climbed over, around, or through in your journey? Are there roads that you have barricaded or blocked? Can you find a picture to represent these?

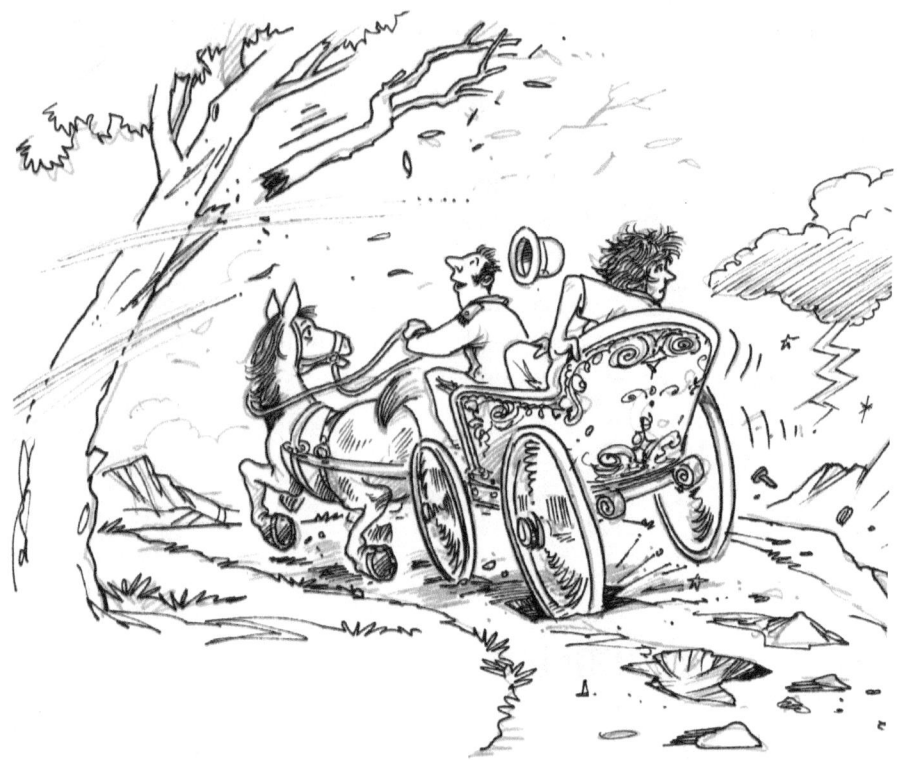

Doubts, Fears, Worries, and Uncertainties

There are three types of worries on a timeline: yesterday's, today's, and tomorrow's.

1. Yesterday's worries are about things that you have said or done, and you fret about the consequences, wishing you could have the moment back to redo it.
2. Tomorrow's worries are about what you would like or not like to happen. With tomorrow's worries, you plan and plot the good or

bad scenarios that might possibly occur. The more inventive you are, the greater possibility you have of creating tomorrow's worries. This is because the little of what may possibly occur tomorrow arises from your imagination. Most worries about the future never take place.

3. Today's worries are in the immediate twenty-four hours or less. They are full of anxious doubts and fears. They hold a feeling of danger from our do-or-die programming, although the event may not be life-threatening at all.

> My Aunt Nonie's favourite saying:
>
> Yesterday is a Cancelled Cheque,
> Tomorrow a Promissory Note,
> Today is Cash on Hand,
> Spend it Wisely.

When I was young, my mother explained what happens if you worry by telling me the story of Kim by Rudyard Kipling. What I remember of what she told me goes like this.

> There once was an old man and a young boy who lived in ancient India. The old man's name was Sartamus, and the boy was called Kim. Kim's parents had died and left him orphaned, and so he had to fend for himself. He went from village to village in search of leftover food thrown away by others. He would do odd jobs wherever he could in return for something to eat or a place to sleep. Kim grew tired of living from day to day, always in search of food and a place to make his home. He questioned the meaning of his life. He wondered, *Why do we as human beings travel through our lives in search of a mere existence? Why are things as difficult as they are? Do we make them so ourselves, or is it just meant to be that we must struggle as we do?*

Kim decided to go search for the answers to the questions on the reason and meaning of his life.

One day he met an old man travelling the same road. The old man was carrying on his back a large, covered, woven basket. Kim quickly caught up to the man and began to walk alongside him. To Kim it looked as if the man carried all his belongings in the basket as it bent him over with its weight.

"What is in your basket that makes it so heavy?" Kim asked Sartamus. "I am young and strong. I would be happy to carry it for you."

The tired old man answered, "It is nothing you could carry for me. This is something I must carry for myself. One day soon enough, you will walk your own road and carry a basket as weighted as mine."

The old man consented to have Kim walk alongside him, and together they travelled many miles. Kim often asked Sartamus questions about life and man's existence. "Why must men always work for never-ending daily needs? Is there nothing more to life then this?" Kim did not get from Sartamus any satisfying answers, nor could he find out what treasure of such great weight was in the basket the old man carried.

Sometimes late at night, when Kim would pretend to be asleep, he would hear the old man sorting through the contents of his basket, talking to himself as he did. Some mornings the basket seemed lighter, or was it that the old man was less weary? Kim looked on the ground around the fire where the old man had done his sorting but found no clue as to the basket's treasure.

The Carriage Ride

One day Sartamus could walk no more, and he lay down to rest for the last time. In their last few hours together, he told Kim his secret, and at the same time, the solution to why men toil vainly.

"In this basket," Sartamus said, "are all of the things I believed about myself—every doubt, fear, every worry, and uncertainty. On my journey I have collected them and have carried their weight on my back. Without these, I could have gone so far, but they held me back. I could have lived a life of the dreams I saw in my mind, but they were a millstone around my neck. They have brought me here, travelling the road and never reaching my goals." The old man closed his eyes and lay down with the basket still strapped on his back. Kim carefully freed Sartamus from the basket and gave him a proper funeral in Indian fashion.

Before Kim went to sleep that night, he untied the leather straps that held the cover of Sartamus's woven basket and looked inside. The basket that had weighted old Sartamus down for so long was empty.

The next morning, Kim picked up the basket and tied it on his own back. He vowed then that at the end of each day when he did his sorting he would throw out the pebbles of doubt or the grains of uncertainty that he had collected during the day. He did not want to become as weighed down as Sartamus had with an accumulation of discouraging thoughts, beliefs, and ideas about himself. He wanted to travel his road unencumbered so that he could enjoy each precious day and reach whatever goals he set for himself.

Many people like Sartamus do not carry just today's worries with them but yesterday's and tomorrow's as well. Are you one of these people?

Jacquie Robinson

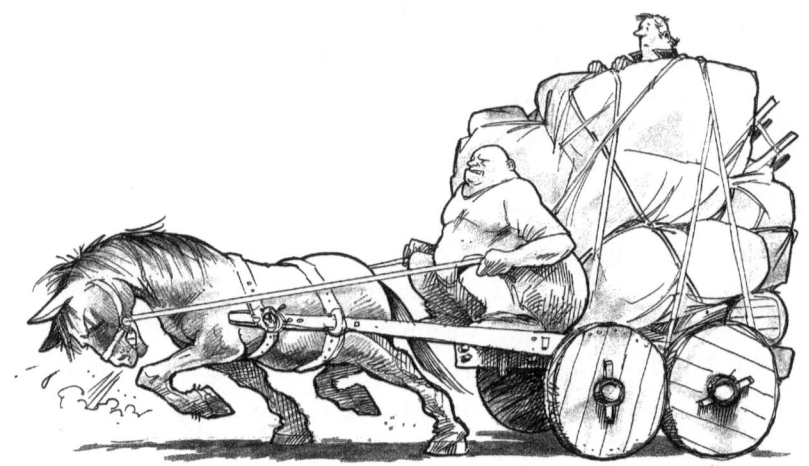

The Carriage Ride

EXERCISE 18: DOUBTS, FEARS, AND WORRIES

What doubts, fears, worries, and uncertainties are you carrying as baggage? Are they yesterday's, today's, or tomorrow's? Fill in the table below.

Doubts, Fears, and Worries		
Yesterday	Today	Tomorrow

Read back over the list. Circle the things you would like to keep, and put a line through those that you can stop carrying with you.

Sometimes other people will attempt to have you help carry their baggage. You do not have to carry baggage—yours or anyone else's. If someone tries to put their doubts, fears, worries, or concerns onto you, simply refuse to take them on.

Significant Events, Turning Points, and Changes of Direction

It is through the stories you tell yourself that you recollect significant events. These can become turning points and changes of direction during the ride of your life. The following are a series of tools based on the art of storytelling: the famous five Ws—what, when, where, who, and why. Often it is not the event that affects us the most but the story and the meaning that we derive from it.

> Imagine that you have on your chest a tape recorder. Over your heart (on your left side) is the record button, on the other side of your chest is eject, and in the centre is erase. When someone gives you a compliment, record it by pushing the button over your heart. When someone attempts to give you a worry, concern, doubt, or fear, simply push reject. Use the erase button for all unwanted worries that you have recorded in the past and are now replaying. I have noticed that people often find it easier to reject compliments than to accept them. Do not hesitate to push that button over your heart and acknowledge it with a simple complement, thank you!

Exercise 19: The Famous Five Ws

1. What: What happened?

The question of what opens up avenues of exploration.

Question	Answer
What happened?	
What was its purpose?	
What was its value?	

What category does it belong to?
    Good?
    Bad?
    Fun?
    Sad?	

What was its part in a larger picture?	
What were its parts?	
What was its history?	
What were its causes?	
What were its effects?	
What was its duration?	
What was its meaning to you?	

2. When: When did this happen?

The question of when events occur in a moment of time. All questions looking at the time of the event are 'when' questions, even though they may not start with when.

Question	Answer
When did the event you described above occur?	
What happened before this?	

Question	Answer
What happened after this?	
Will it happen again?	
What else was happening at the same time?	
How often does it happen?	
Has it happened previously?	
What conditions must be met in order for it to happen?	
How would this have been different if it had happened at another time?	
How is it similar to things that have happened at other times?	
How long did it last?	

3. *Where:* Where did this event occur?

Everything is somewhere, and describing that place permits you to discover the sights, sounds, smells, and the whole sense of the event. Descriptive detail invites you to re-enter the scene imaginatively and to look around. Use the question of where to orientate yourself. This helps you to know not only where the thing happened but also what this place was like for you at that time. Remember that if the event occurred when you were a child, the places and people may appear much bigger, scarier, and larger than life.

Question	Answer
Where did the event occur? Describe the place in as much detail as possible	
Can you imagine the place where you stood? If you can, stand there, look out and describe what you see?	

Can you focus in on all the minute details of where you were, then pull back, to take in the larger scene?	

> *My sister, Joy, and I always talked of how much fun we had playing on a huge hill beside our house. We spent hours in the summer, rolling down it. And in the winter, we went sliding on our toboggan. Recently, when visiting Canada with my husband, I took him to see my home in Ailsa Craig where I grew up. It was quite a surprise to see the hill that I remembered as being so big was not a hill at all, but just a small culvert that ran alongside the road next to our house. I realised then just how big the world is in the eyes of a child.*

4. *Who:* Who was involved in this event?

You can answer this question with one word—for example, Mum, Dad, Grandpa, Grandma—but this gives you only a superficial description. Filling in their background, their personality, and physical and character descriptions provides a complete, three-dimensional picture.

Question	Answer
Who was involved in the event? Describe the people as you remember them.	
What do you know about them?	
Can you step into their shoes and describe the event from their eyes?	

5. *Why:* Why was this event important in your journey?

Why asks you to look for the meanings that you have given to these events. Some therapists say that "why" should be avoided as it is a bottomless pit of imagination and projection. I believe the question of why can help you develop a fuller understanding of yourself. The better you understand yourself, the better your chances of living your life entirely in your own chosen way. Making sense of why can help you choose whether you want to do it again.

Question	**Answer**
Why is this event important in your journey?	
Why does it come to mind when others don't?	
Why did this happen?	
Can you identify a cause?	
How many other causes are possible?	
Which causes are more or less important to you now?	
Were the results intentional or accidental?	
How might the event be seen in a new light?	

· · · · · ·

Dr. Gagné a psychiatrist I worked with for many years in Sherbrooke, Quebec, used to say:

"It is not only important to take note of 'what' a person is telling you but also keep in mind 'why' are they telling 'you' this and what are they leaving out?"

The Carriage Ride

Exercise 20: Using the Model to Master Your Life

The Ride of Your Life model provides the possibility of distinguishing your thoughts from your feelings. Your thoughts about a certain situation lead to your emotional response. The trick is to become aware of what it is you are telling yourself. Here is how to do it.

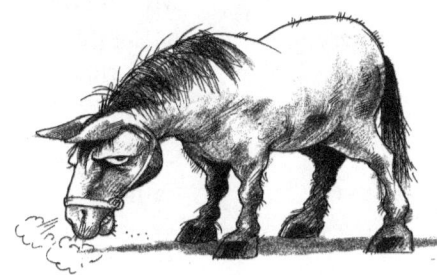 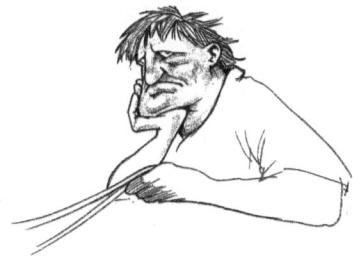

1. Stop—Stand or sit still. Be present to this moment of your existence using your senses to experience life for and by yourself.
2. Breathe in and out slowly. Perceive all the different aromas in the air by inhaling through your nose.
3. Listen to the sounds around you. Discover their sources.
4. Look at your surroundings, and detect all the colours, shapes, and shades. Focus in on all the minute details you can and then pull back, taking in the largest, full picture possible.
5. Feel the warmth and/or coolness of the air around you. Touch all the different textures that you can find (only those politely permissible, of course).
6. Now think of your past and from where you have come to get to this exact point in time.
7. Describe the taste of your life. Do you discern it as sweet, sour, salty, spicy, bland, and/or bitter?
8. Determine your emotional state. Use the following list to write down as many feelings as you can detect.

	Bashful	Depressed	Embarrassed
Alienated	Bored	Determined	Enthusiastic
Angry	Cautious	Disappointed	Envious
Annoyed	Confident	Discouraged	Ecstatic
Anxious	Confused	Disgusted	Excited
Apathetic	Curious	Exhausted	
Fearful	Happy	Innocent	Mischievous
Frightened	Helpless	Interested	Miserable
Frustrated	Hopeful	Irritated	Negative
Good	Hostile	Jealous	Numb
Guilty	Humiliated	Lonely	Optimistic
	Hurt	Loved	Pained
	Hysterical	Lovestruck	
Paranoid	Sad	Surprised	Unloved
Peaceful	Satisfied	Suspicious	Withdrawn
Proud	Shocked	Shy	
Puzzled	Sorry	Thoughtful	
Regretful	Stubborn	Trapped	
Relieved	Sure	Undecided	

9. To discover the connection between your feelings and your thoughts, notice the thoughts that come into your mind the moment you say, "I feel sad," or, "happy," or, "jealous," and so on, "because." Remember the "because" is the entity that you are holding responsible for your feelings. Having uncovered this thought, you can choose to keep it if you want to or let it go. You choose your thoughts; they do not choose you.

10. Check your body; do you have any tense or tight muscles, aches, or pains in any areas; an upset stomach; are you hot and flushed or cold and clammy?

11. You have now detected your emotions, your thoughts, and your physical state in the present moment. Breathe in deeply, relax, and experience your life. Take a moment of your time to just "be" with yourself. This is a unique moment in the ride of your life. Cherish it.

12. Your future road of life lays ahead of you in any direction you choose to take from this point forward. Let your mind wander to all the possibilities you want to take. See these as roads you can choose to explore.
13. Now, choose the road of your life. Not what you think you should do but what you would prefer for yourself. Where do you want to go? What do you want to do? Make a plan to do it.
14. See yourself being there. Step into your future of your making. This is the ride you choose for your life.

Conclusion

Being the master of the ride of your life requires that you get all your carriage parts to work together. When working well, your carriage, horse, driver, and master are a team working harmoniously, enabling you to get where you want to go.

With the Ride of Your Life model, you have a means to understanding yourself as a human being. This workbook has little value if you only read it and then put it back on the bookshelf. What I hope you will do is use your new knowledge to help live a most fulfilling ride of your life!

...

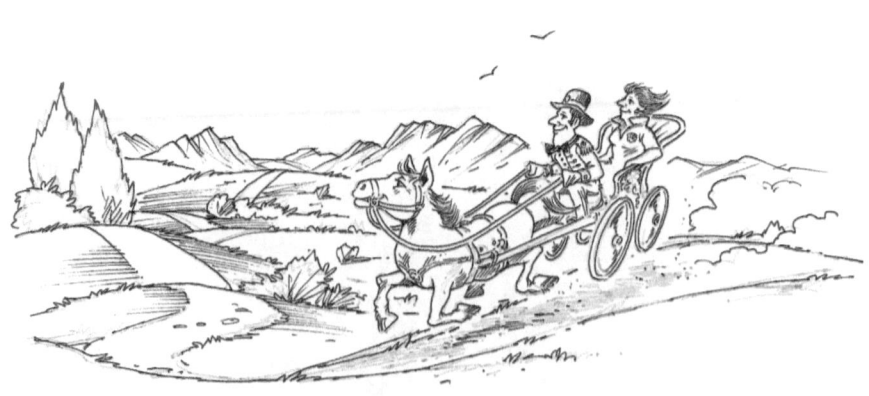

The End

NOTES

Now that you have read The Carriage Ride and understand the Ride of Your Life model it is time to put the theory into practice.

Yogi Berra once said *"In theory there is no difference between theory and practice. In practice there is."*

In the Notes section write down how you are applying what you have learnt from The Carriage Ride in the ride of your life.

My Example

I have found The Carriage Ride Workbook with its Ride of Your Life Model helping me appreciate my input into my life's adventure. I know that I am happiest when I am learning and discovering something new. So I made a picture anxiety scale using the parts of the Ride of Your Life Model to help identify anxiety levels. When I provide individual therapy, run group therapy, give workshops, and lectures or present at conferences on The Carriage Ride workbook, I share the Picture Anxiety Scale and explain how to use it. I am collecting feedback on the Carriage Ride Workbook and the Picture Anxiety scale to learn how helpful they are. This research is my present journey. My future goal is the sequel to this book on sharing the road of your life with others.

REFERENCES

Berne, Eric. (1964). *Games People Play: The Basic Handbook of Transactional Analysis* New York. Grove Press. (http://www.ericberne.com/).

Von Oech, Roger. (1992). *Creative Whack Pack (Cards)*. Creative Whack Company. (http://www.creativewhack.com/product.php?productid=64).

Berra, Yogi. Yogi Berra Quotes (http://www.brainyquote.com/quotes/quotes/y/yogiberra141506.html)

About the Artist

All cartoons are by the Flinders Ranges, Australia,–based artist George Grainger Aldridge. He usually paints huge, beautiful landscapes of the Adnyamathanha country in the northern mountains and portraits of those who live in them. For the work of George Grainger Aldridge, contact him at <u>aldridge_george@yahoo.com.au</u>.

www.ingramcontent.com/pod-product-compliance
Lightning Source LLC
Chambersburg PA
CBHW021949200526
45163CB00018B/1950